LIVING AT HOME WITH DEMENTIA

RICHARD STOKES

authorHOUSE

AuthorHouse™
1663 Liberty Drive
Bloomington, IN 47403
www.authorhouse.com
Phone: 1 (800) 839-8640

Published by AuthorHouse 06/05/2019

ISBN: 978-1-7283-1284-2 (sc)
ISBN: 978-1-7283-1283-5 (e)

Print information available on the last page.

DEDICATION

This Handbook is dedicated to the harvest of friends
God sent to us who spent much time with Margaret
during her struggle with Dementia at home.

INTRODUCTION

Dementia is an ever-changing disease that will require a lot of hard work on your part. Therefore, it's important to keep yourself healthy so you can deal with what you are to meet down the road with this ever-changing disease. Making the decision to keep a loved one at home with a terminal disease, as opposed to a nursing home or assisted living is a difficult decision to make, one that I pondered for a considerable time before deciding to keep Margaret, my wife of fifty-four years at home to care for her.

If you decide to keep your loved one at home you must commit yourself to hard work and a great deal of patience and understanding. I will always be grateful for the assistance of Heartland who provided someone to bathe Margaret and a regular nurse to help monitor her vital signs.

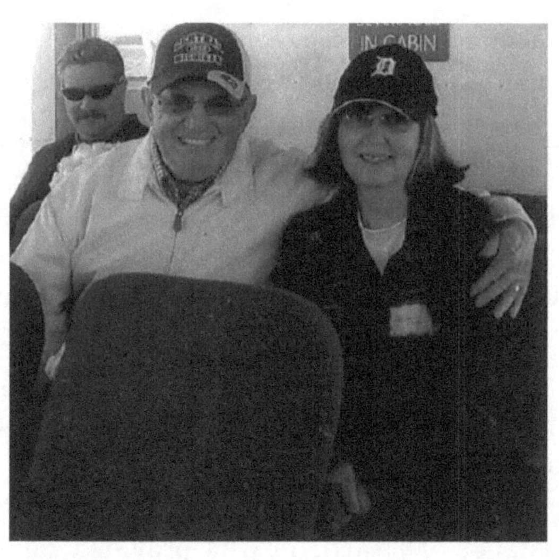
IN CABIN

CREATING A POSITIVE ATMOSPHERE

Play soft music when a person is either sitting up in a chair or even after they have gone to be to help them to relax. Bring out pictures of the family and let the person talk about them as much as they can. Talk about the good old days and memories as long as it does not cause the person to become agitated. Each person is different and you will be the professional at knowing what things will make them happy and what will not go over well. Share this information with other caregivers.

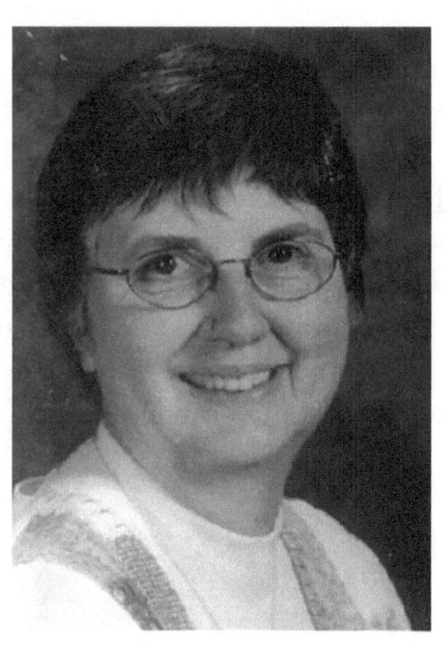

MOVING A PERSON

Bend at the knees and straighten up by using your thigh muscles. Keep your back straight, and don't bend at the waist. Space your feet comfortably apart to gain support. Use a transfer or easy belt. This allows you to have a good grip on the person without grabbing their arms. To help move the person wrap the transfer belt around the person's waist and slide him or her to the edge of the chair or bed. Face the person and place your hands under the belt on either side of his or her waist. Then bend your knees and pull up by using your thigh muscles to raise the person from a seated to a standing position.

Remember to cue them about each step as you do it and tell them you need them to help you. "Okay Margaret, now I need you to push up with your legs when I count to three...one, two, three, and push!" This helps them remember to do what you need them to do.

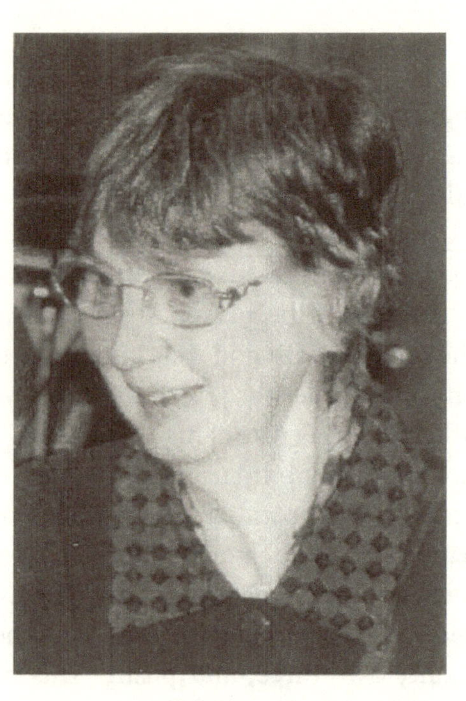

MEDICINES

Make certain all medicines are safely out of reach of your loved one at all times. Use child safe caps if possible. If your loved one is having difficulty swallowing pills cut the pills in half so the person won't choke. A pill cutter can be purchased at the local pharmacy and make the pill easier to administer. Difficulty taking meds is something that should be reported to a doctor or nurse as ability to swallow declines.

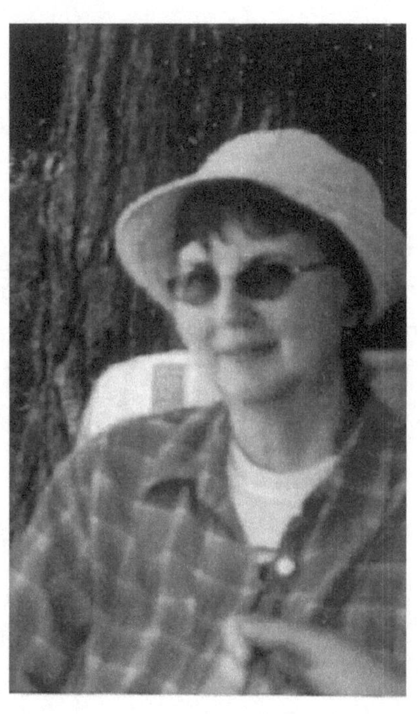

TRAVELING BY AUTOMOBILE

Make certain all the doors are locked to prevent the person from falling out of the automobile. Make certain the person is sitting straight up in the seat so that the airbag will be properly engaged. Always help the person out of the car to help prevent falls from occurring.

Report any declines in ability to walk, near falls, or actual falls to the doctor or nurse as they may help come up with ideas and equipment to keep the person safe and at the highest level of functioning as long as possible.

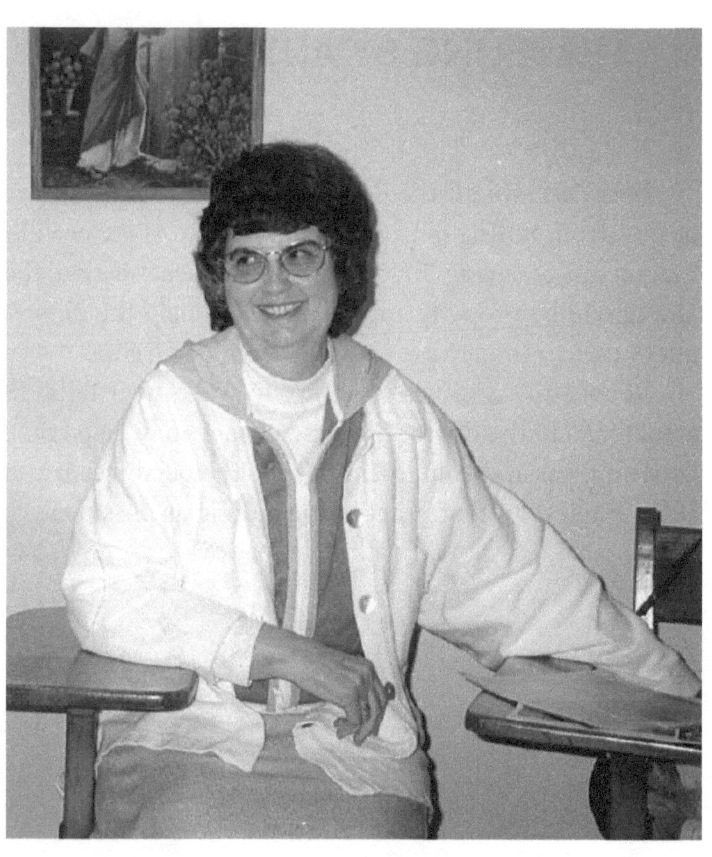

DRESSING

Lay out clothes in the order the person should put them on. Hand the person one thing at a time. Put away some clothes in another room to help reduce the number of choices. Allow the person to do as much as possible for the themselves, assisting only as needed.

Spiritual activities. Involve the person in attending church services. Play religious or other music that is important to the person. Let them browse through photo albums or look at newspapers or magazines to reminisce avoiding troublesome news on TV or in the paper as it could cause agitation or fear.

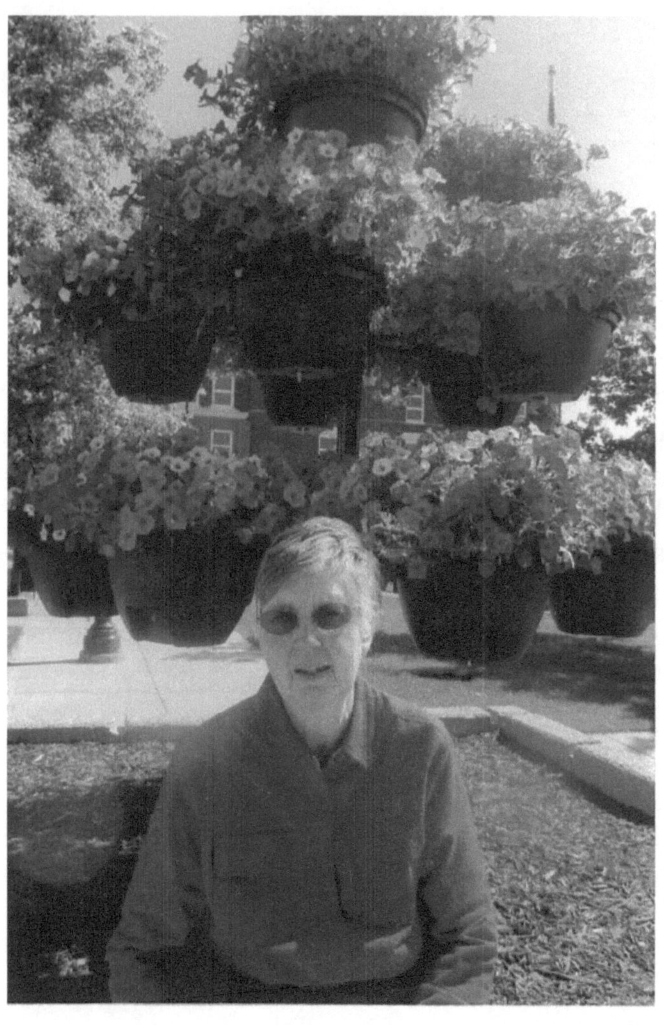

SWALLOWING PROBLEM

Cut food into small pieces and make it soft enough to eat. Use a blender to grind food. Don't use straws. It may cause a swallowing problem. Limit the use of milk as it may catch in the throat. Give the person cold drinks because they are easy to swallow.

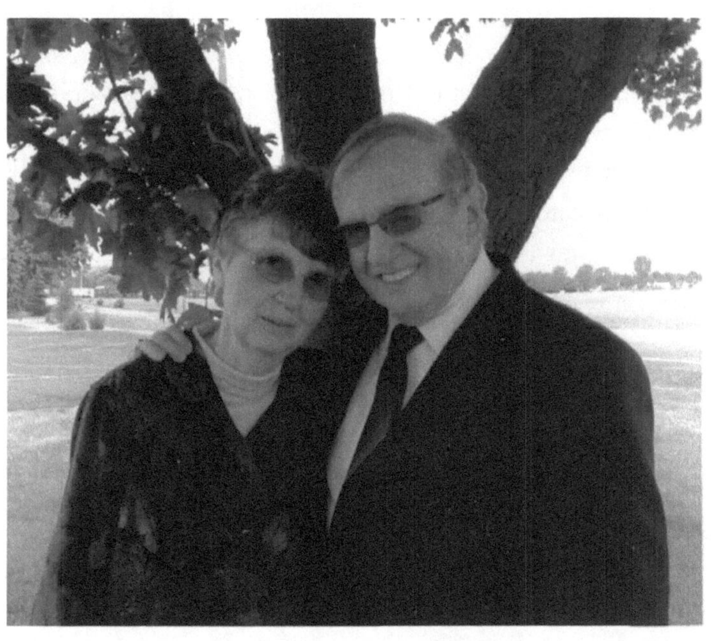

CLOTHING

Lay out morning and night time clothing. Ask the person if they need assistance in taking off or putting on clothing. Whenever possible let the person choose the clothing to wear but limit choices to two or three to not overwhelm them. Even if the color or material don't match, if the person is happy about their selection don't force them to wear something they're unhappy with. Make sure they have clean and unstained clothing to maintain their dignity when in public.

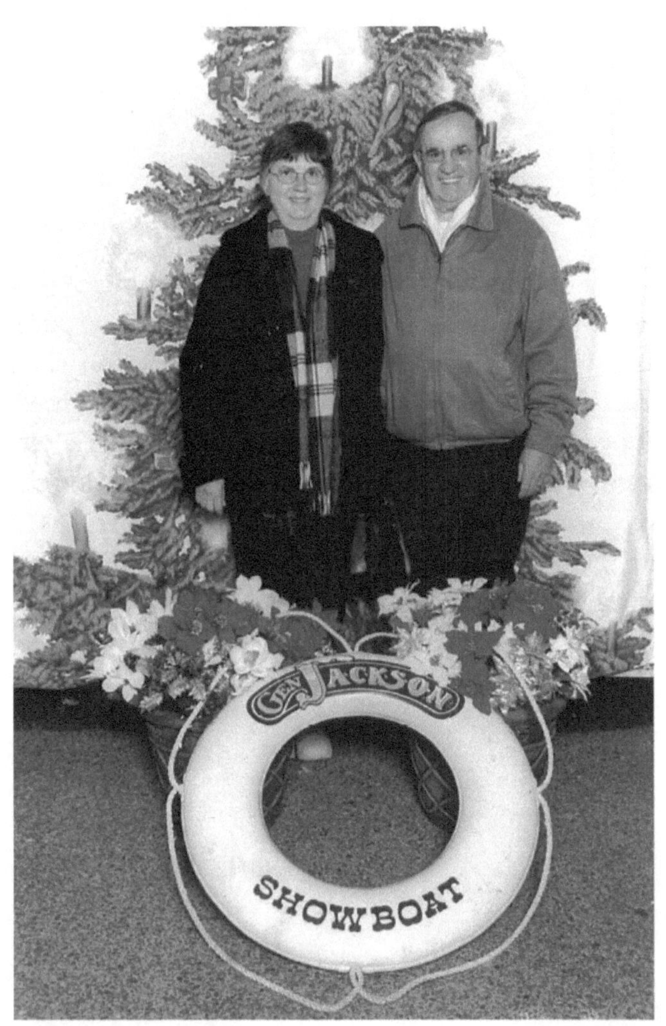
Gen Jackson
SHOWBOAT

VISITORS

When your loved one is staying at home he or she will have visitors from time to time. Ask visitors to keep their visit short so the person doesn't tire. Lengthy visits will tire the person and can cause them to become agitated. As dementia progresses, it is normal for the person to become sleepier and doze off and on throughout the day. Sometimes dementia patients suffer from insomnia and aren't able to sleep at night and then want to sleep all day. Report this to a doctor or nurse for assistance in helping the person get into a good sleep pattern. Prolonged periods of sleeplessness can lead to increased negative behaviors and even Psychosis if left untreated.

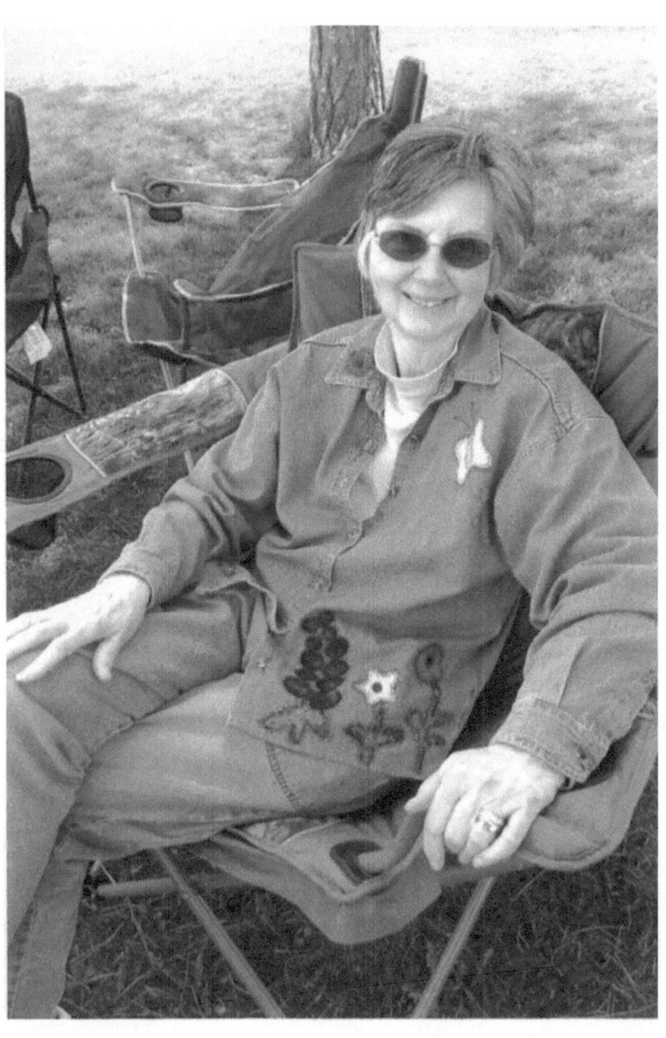

COMMUNICATION

It is important to connect with your loved one. The disease progression can cause words, sentences, and thoughts to get jumbled or confused. Often the person will say illogical things. It is best to not correct them because they may become frustrated, angry, or even fearful.

Speak with a soft voice and try and keep eye contact as long as you can. Use every opportunity to hold the person's hand both in talking and just sitting with them. Try to keep the person involved by listening to their ideas when expressed. If things become too much for you, you may want to leave the room for a while. Be patient with the person. Pray and ask God to give your the right words to use when communicating with your loved one.

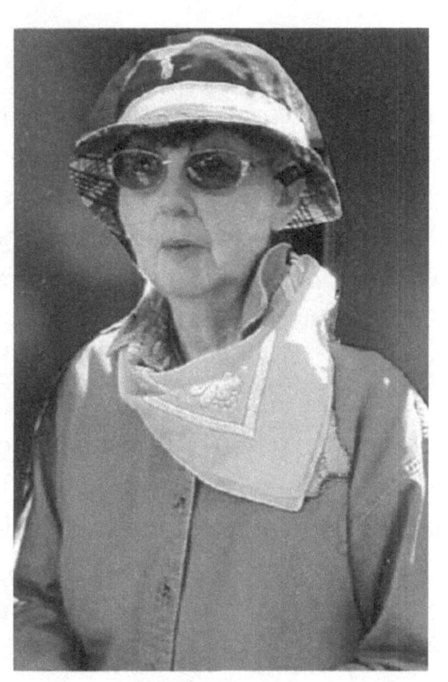

CHANGE IN BEHAVIOR

When changes in behavior come remember the changes can be caused by medicines, pain, poor eyesight or hearing, or general fatigue. When you aren't sure what's going on contact your nurse or a doctor. Keep things simple. Have a daily routine so the person can keep track of when things will happen. Use humor when you can. Ask for their help. For example, "let's set the table together."

SLEEP PROBLEMS

Have the person go to bed at the same time each night. Put small lights in the bedroom and hallway. Margret was a blessing because she never wandered around the house or tried to leave. Some people are less fortunate than I and must monitor activity constantly. Give the person something to for them to take to bed such as a favorite teddy bear, etc. Often the familiar item can provide comfort when disoriented at night. Always make sure the person is safe and can't reach anything that could be used to hurt anyone or themselves. (Ex. Lock up chemicals and sharp knives, etc.)

WANDERING

Margret never attempted to leave the house, however, I did have a necklace made with her name and address on it, just in case. I let all neighbors know of her condition so they could be aware of the situation. I also put a sign on the street which said, "caution: dementia person lives here."

THE FAMILY

Family deal with the loss of memory and abilities differently. Some want to see the person a lot and some find it too difficult. You need to keep the family informed about your love one's progress. Encourage them to visit as often as they can. Tell them about the disease and how things will change possibly from day to day. Share books about the disease to help them understand what is happening to their friend.

HOME SAFETY

Make certain you have carbon monoxide and smoke alarms in the kitchen and in all bedrooms. Child proof plugs should be installed for any unused electrical outlets. Keep all emergency phone numbers handy, including poison control. Make certain all medicines are carefully put away. Lock up all guns, scissors, and knives or anything else that might be harmful. Put signs on things that may prove to be harmful as a warning. Sometimes using red stop signs will signal the person to not enter an area that is someone else's bedroom for instance. Remove throw rugs as they might become slippery. Also, watch for spills on the floor. Purchase shoe and slippers with good traction to prevent slip and fall accidents and remove clutter from walkways.

HEALTHY EATING

Buy healthy foods and/or fruits, vegetables, and whole grain products. Be sure to buy food that the person enjoys and is able to eat. Buy food that is easy to prepare. Always serve meals at the same time each day. Offer just one food at a time instead of filling the plate with too many things. Often people with dementia have difficulty swallowing and it can worsen over time. Update your nurse or doctor if you see changes in ability to chew or swallow.

BATHING

Never leave a confused or frail person alone in the tub or shower. Make sure the water is not too hot or cold. Use a hand held showerhead. Use a rubber bath mat and put safety bars in the tub. Use a sturdy shower chair in the tub or shower. Before a bath or shower, be gentle and respectful. Tell the person what you are going to do step by step. Put a towel over the person's shoulders or lap. If the person becomes upset talk about something else. If the person has difficulty getting in and out of the bathtub do a sponge bath instead. A non-slip bath mat on the floor outside the tub is also recommended.

This Handbook is not all inclusive. However, it will help to keep you focused as you care for your loved one at home with Dementia. Although I miss Margaret greatly, I know she is now in a better place free of pain and suffering.

I'm grateful to have experienced the opportunity of sharing Margaret's final days with her. I'm also extremely grateful for the involvement of Heartland Hospice and their team of professionals. I owe them a great deal and will always cherish the opportunity I had to work with them and watch their tender care of Margaret. Thank you for reading this Handbook. Remember you don't have do everything alone. There are many resources available to you.

RESOURCES

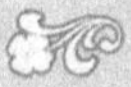

If you are interested in learning more, here is a sampling of resources.
Some of these are also listed at the end of most chapters.

AARP
1-888-687-2277 (toll-free)
1-877-342-2277 (español/línea gratis)
1-877-434-7598 (TTY/toll-free)
member@aarp.org (email)
www.aarp.org

Aging with Dignity
1-888-594-7437 (toll-free)
fivewishes@agingwithdignity.org
(email)
www.agingwithdignity.org

Alzheimer's Association
1-800-272-3900 (toll-free)
1-866-403-3073 (TTY/toll-free)
info@alz.org (email)
www.alz.org

Alzheimer's Foundation of America
1-866-232-8484 (toll-free)
info@alzfdn.org (email)
www.alzfdn.org

**American Academy of Hospice
and Palliative Medicine**
info@aahpm.org (email)
www.palliativedoctors.org

American Academy of Pain Medicine
1-847-375-4731
info@painmed.org (email)
www.painmed.org

American Bar Association
1-800-285-2221 (toll-free)
www.americanbar.org/contactus
(email form)
www.americanbar.org

American Board of Wound Management
1-202-457-8408
info@abwmcertified.org (email)
www.aawm.org

American Geriatrics Society
Health in Aging Foundation
1-800-563-4916 (toll-free)
info@healthinaging.org (email)
www.healthinaging.org

American Music Therapy Association
1-301-589-3300
info@musictherapy.org (email)
www.musictherapy.org

Association for Conflict Resolution
1-202-780-5999
admin@acrnet.org (email)
www.acrnet.org

CaringBridge
www.CaringBridge.org

CaringInfo
(See National Hospice and Palliative Care Organization)

Center for Elder Care and Advanced Illness
Altarum Institute
1-202-776-5100
eldercare@altarum.org (email)
www.altarum.org/cecai

Center for Practical Bioethics
1-800-344-3829 (toll-free)
info@practicalbioethics.org (email)
www.practicalbioethics.org

Centers for Medicare and Medicaid Services
1-800-633-4227 (toll-free)
1-877-486-2048 (TTY/toll-free)
www.medicare.gov

Center to Advance Palliative Care
1-212-201-2670
capc@mssm.edu (email)
www.getpalliativecare.org

Department of Veterans Affairs
Veterans Benefits Administration
Veterans Health Administration
VA benefits:
1-800-827-1000 (toll-free)
To speak with a healthcare benefits counselor:
1-877-222-8387 (toll-free)
www.va.gov

Donate Life America
1-804-377-3580
donatelifeamerica@donatelife.net (email)
www.donatelife.net

Education in Palliative and End-of-life Care (EPEC)
1-312-503-3732
info@epec.net (email)
www.epec.net

Eldercare Locator
1-800-677-1116 (toll-free)
www.eldercare.gov

Family Caregiver Alliance
1-800-445-8106 (toll-free)
info@caregiver.org (email)
www.caregiver.org

Federal Trade Commission
1-877-382-4357 (toll-free)
www.ftc.gov

Growth House
1-415-863-3045
info@growthhouse.org (email)
www.growthhouse.org

Hospice Association of America
National Association for Home
Care and Hospice
1-202-546-4759
www.nahc.org/HAA

**Hospice and Palliative Nurses
Association**
1-412-787-9301
hpna@hpna.org (email)
http://hpna.advancingexpertcare.org

Hospice Foundation of America
1-800-854-3402 (toll-free)
info@hospicefoundation.org (email)
www.hospicefoundation.org
www.hospicedirectory.org

Hospice Net
info@hospicenet.org (email)
www.hospicenet.org

The Living Bank
1-800-528-2971 (toll-free)
info@livingbank.org (email)
www.livingbank.org

National Alliance for Caregiving
1-301-718-8444
info@caregiving.org (email)
www.caregiving.org

**National Alliance for
Hispanic Health**
1-866-783-2645 (English and
Spanish; toll-free)
membership@healthyamericas.org
(email)
www.hispanichealth.org

National Cancer Institute
1-800-422-6237 (toll-free)
cancergovstaff@mail.nih.gov (email)
www.cancer.gov
www.cancer.gov/cancertopics/
factsheet/support/end-of-life-care

**National Hospice and Palliative
Care Organization**
1-800-658-8898 (toll-free)
caringinfo@nhpco.org (email)
www.caringinfo.org
www.nhpco.org

**National Institute of Nursing
Research**
1-301-496-0207
info@ninr.nih.gov (email)
www.ninr.nih.gov

National Library of Medicine
www.medlineplus.gov
Search for:
"Advance Directives"
"Bereavement"
"End-of-Life Issues"
"Hospice Care"
"Organ Donation"
"Pain"

OrganDonor.gov
Health Resources and Services
Administration
U.S. Department of Health and
Human Services
donation@hrsa.gov (email)
www.organdonor.gov

**Physician Orders for Life-Sustaining
Treatment Paradigm (POLST)**
1-503-494-4463
info@polst.org (email)
www.polst.org

PostHope
http://posthope.org

PREPARE
1-415-735-1106
info@prepareforyourcare.org (email)
www.prepareforyourcare.org

Society of Critical Care Medicine
1-847-827-6869
info@sccm.org (email)
www.myicucare.org/Pages/default.aspx

Social Security Administration
1-800-772-1213 (toll-free)
1-800-325-0778 (TTY/toll-free)
www.socialsecurity.gov

U.S. Department of Health and Human Services
www.alzheimers.gov

Visiting Nurse Associations of America
1-888-866-8773 (toll-free)
vnaa@vnaa.org (email)
www.vnaa.org

Well Spouse Association
1-800-838-0879 (toll-free)
info@wellspouse.org (email)
www.wellspouse.org

What Matters Now
www.whatmattersnow.org

For more information on health and aging, contact:

National Institute on Aging Information Center
P.O. Box 8057
Gaithersburg, MD 20898-8057
1-800-222-2225 (toll-free)
1-800-222-4225 (TTY/toll-free)
niaic@nia.nih.gov (email)
www.nia.nih.gov

To order publications (in English or Spanish) or sign up for regular email alerts about new publications and other information from the NIA, go to www.nia.nih.gov/health.

Visit www.nihseniorhealth.gov, a senior-friendly website from the National Institute on Aging and the National Library of Medicine. This website has health and wellness information for older adults, including information about end of life care. Special features make it simple to use. For example, you can click on a button to make the type larger.

To learn more about Alzheimer's disease, contact NIA's ADEAR Center at:
Alzheimer's Disease Education and Referral (ADEAR) Center
1-800-438-4380 (toll-free)
adear@nia.nih.gov (email)
www.nia.nih.gov/alzheimers

Resources

For more information on disorders or research programs funded by the
National Institute of Neurological Disorders and Stroke or the National
Institute on Aging, please contact:

National Institute of Neurological Disorders and Stroke
BRAIN
1-800-352-9424 (toll-free)
braininfo@ninds.nih.gov
www.ninds.nih.gov

National Institute on Aging
Alzheimer's and related Dementias Education and Referral
(ADEAR) Center
1-800-438-4380 (toll-free)
adear@nia.nih.gov
www.alzheimers.gov

Information on dementia also is available from the following
organizations:

Alzheimer's Association
1-800-272-3900 (toll-free)
1-866-403-3073 (TTY/toll-free)
info@alz.org
www.alz.org

Alzheimer's Drug Discovery Foundation
1-212-901-8000
info@alzdiscovery.org
www.alzdiscovery.org

Alzheimer's Foundation of America
1-866-232-8484 (toll-free)
info@alzfdn.org
www.alzfdn.org

Association for Frontotemporal Degeneration
1-866-507-7222 (toll-free)
info@theaftd.org
www.theaftd.org

The Bluefield Project to Cure Frontotemporal Dementia
rodney.pearlman@bluefieldproject.org
www.bluefieldproject.org

BrightFocus Foundation
1-800-437-2423 (toll-free)
info@brightfocus.org
www.brightfocus.org/alzheimers

Lewy Body Dementia Association
1-404-975-2322
1-844-311-0587 (toll-free LBD Caregiver Link)
lbda@lbda.org
www.lbda.org

National Institute of Mental Health
1-866-615-6464 (toll-free)
1-866-415-8051 (TTY/toll-free)
nimhinfo@nih.gov
www.nimh.nih.gov

National Organization for Rare Disorders
1-800-999-6673 (toll-free Patient Services)
orphan@rarediseases.org
www.rarediseases.org